HOMEMADE HAND SANITIZER

I0504464

MARGARET GREY

© Copyright 2020 All rights reserved.

Table of Contents

HAND DISINFECTION

Grab it - wipe it - spray it - rub it. It is the hand disinfection boogie. Hand disinfection is a popular method and can be used in wheelbarrows, banks, schools, and other public places where hands can touch other people's hands. And you don't know where those hands were before. Just the thought lets you grab the

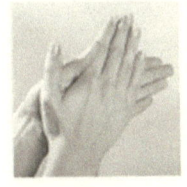 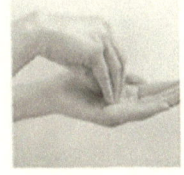 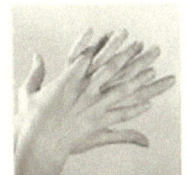

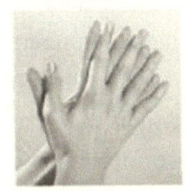 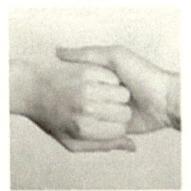 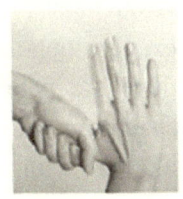

next available hand sanitizer that could very well be in your pocket, jacket, or handbag. The use of hand disinfectants prevents pathogens, virus bugs, and bacteria from sneezing, wheezing, and sometimes causing nausea on us humans and our children. Good or bad, we are a germicidal society. The realization that microorganisms cause illness and even death is one of the more beneficial findings in medicine. The question in the minds and lips of some is: have we gone too far? The idea here is - yes, we have. Germ phobia can be both physically and emotionally unhealthy. This has been demonstrated by the development of seriously lethal antibiotic-resistant bacteria and the stress that some people experience by avoiding germs - A constant burden of disinfecting every corner of the environment.

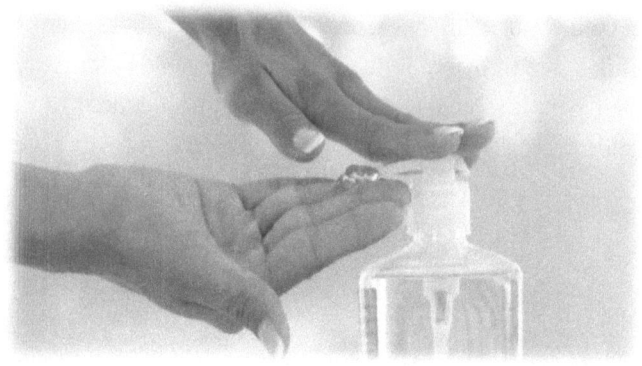

Awareness is good, but delusions to the extent of exaggeration are not. When it comes to hand sanitizers, there are both the good and the bad. One argument against the use of hand sanitizers is that their use may interfere with the development of adaptive immunity in children. Adaptive immunity is a function of the immune system that creates protection against parasitic microorganisms that have previously infected the body. In other words, it's good for your children to get sick. This protects them later in life. It is questionable whether the use of a hand disinfectant has a strong negative impact on adaptive immunity. Research shows that the use of hand disinfectants reduces sick days in schoolchildren, but it is not clear whether this will reduce the number of diseases that children develop during childhood.

The first-hand disinfectant available on the market was a gel that contained alcohol and still does today. Over time, studies came out that showed that alcohol-based hand sanitizers were actually bad for your hands. You see, the alcohol causes the skin to become dry and cracked, creating gaps that trap germs. In fact, studies show that the more you use them, the less effective they will be. It has also been reported that we should not use hand disinfectants as these weaken our resistance and reduce our ability to fight germs. They frightened us to think that if we were to rely on hand disinfectants, we would become weak and unable to ward off bad germs. Let us not forget, of course, the Germaphobics, who also contributed to the bad reputation. When we thought of hand disinfectants, images of eccentric, germ-infested people came to mind, which inexorably pumped hand disinfectants into their pale hands. Not a pretty sight. Well, it's time for someone to speak up and save hand sanitizers. It's time to clear up any popular misunderstandings, open our hearts and minds, and bring hand sanitizers back to their rightful place in society.

Here is the scoop: 80% of the germs are transferred by hand, and since hand washing is not always possible, and alcohol-free hand disinfectant is a perfect solution. Imagine you have a personal invisible shield that protects you from germs around the clock? Non-alcoholic hand disinfectants are gentle, safe for the whole family, non-toxic, non-flammable, and do not leave any sticky residue on your hands. The active substance is benzalkonium chloride and has been used extensively by doctors for over 40 years. It is approved for safety and effectiveness in many antiseptic applications, including skin treatments. It is also widely used as a preservative in cosmetics and many over-the-counter products, including nasal sprays for infants. These alcohol-free hand disinfectants kill 99.9% of the germs in less than 15 seconds. We are talking about the malicious germs that cause diseases such as Salmonella, Norwalk virus, E. coli, SARS, bird flu, and more.

If hand washing is not possible, alcohol-free hand disinfectants are the answer. There are portable mini sprays that you can carry in your handbag, briefcase, backpack, computer bag, and bags. Or take one with you when shopping, travelling, flying, driving, or taking the subway. Always keep one "on-hand" (you must have seen one coming) ... keep one at your desk, in the rooms of your house, or in your locker at school. Alcohol-free hand disinfectants are affordable, practical, and can protect you and your family from disease-causing germs. Stop the injustice and spread of germs and get an alcohol-free hand disinfectant today and stay healthy!

Triclosan is an antibacterial, antiviral, and antifungal agent that is used in many consumer products, including hand sanitizers. The evidence is not complete that triclosan is safe for humans. Several scientific studies have been published since the last review of this ingredient. Animal studies have shown that triclosan changes hormone regulation. However, data showing

4

effects on animals does not always mean that the effects on humans have gone one step further. Other studies on bacteria have shown that triclosan helps to make bacteria resistant to antibiotics. "The good thing is, triclosan is not even necessary in a hand disinfectant. The main component of the most effective hand sanitizer is alcohol. For a product to be 99% effective, the content must be at least 60% ethanol (alcohol).

HAND HYGIENE AND HAND DISINFECTANTS

The word hygiene is derived from the ancient Greek goddess. Hygeia, the goddess of healing. Hygiene today is associated with disease prevention and health promotion. The importance of hygiene is generally recognized and evidence-based. Physical contact between people and things is an important means for the transmission of pathogens. Therefore, effective hand hygiene is an important intervention in disease prevention. This is an essential step in the healthcare system, and healthcare workers are regularly trained in hand hygiene procedures. In the community outside of health care, studies have found a link between improvements in hand hygiene and a reduction in infection rates. It is estimated that simply washing your hands could save a million lives a year, and many public health campaigns around the world have had varying degrees of success with "hand hygiene." However, studies show that after washing hands, up to 80% of people keep some pathogenic bacteria on their hands. Washing hands with soap remove the body's own fatty acids from the skin, which can lead to cracked skin, which provides an entry portal for pathogens. In contrast, high-quality hand disinfectants contain additional skincare products such as plasticizers. You don't need water either, which makes it easy and straightforward to use.

Compliance with hand hygiene practices among health professionals has been regularly reviewed and examined. To our knowledge, hand hygiene practices in the general population have rarely been studied. In addition, the effectiveness of various hand disinfectant formulations in reducing bacterial exposure in non-healthcare settings has not been investigated. Many people have the misunderstanding that their immediate surroundings must be sterile. Well, this is only possible in a real aseptic chamber in a laboratory or in certain hospital settings. We live in a natural world full of microorganisms, living things that cannot be seen with the naked eye. Some microorganisms can cause disease, while others can be essential to our environment and well-being. Some microorganisms can cause food spoilage and disease, but many without good bacteria, you will not take your favourite yogurt, sauerkraut, or certain medicines! Cows could not use the grass to produce energy without a good microbial partner. And without good bacteria and fungi, our earth is filled with garden waste and other biological waste. In addition, we must not forget that our normal, healthy body has various external barriers and internal mechanisms (immune system) to fight bacteria unless the number of bacteria is overwhelming. So if we understand and learn how to control or deal with both the good and bad microorganisms in our bodies and in our environment, we can make good use of these microbes. At the same time, it limits the spread of infectious diseases. The goal is to decrease the number of bad bacteria to very low levels so that the body can get rid of its existing immune system.

The body parts of healthy people and animals are hosts to a variety of microbes known as resident microbes. Upon contact with other objects, the body also absorbs other microorganisms called transient microorganisms. For example, a typical human hand can carry 10,000 to 10 million bacteria, some of which are resident and some of which are temporary. If people or animals are sick or infected with certain microbes, the number of microbes can increase.

Skin is not the only host area in the body of bacteria and other microorganisms. Many microorganisms also exist in the intestinal tract of humans and animals. These are known as faecal microorganisms.

A person's hands, arms, or fingers can become contaminated with faecal microorganisms after using the toilet. These have to be removed by mechanical friction when washing with water and soap or destroyed by using antiseptic solutions. Microorganisms from humans and animals can move to the hand, other people, food, and everything that comes into contact with the hand, and vice versa. For this reason, good handwashing is important to reduce harmful microorganisms on our hands and to reduce the risk of spreading harmful microorganisms to others.

ALCOHOL

Pure ethyl alcohol (ethanol) is undoubtedly a better choice than isopropyl alcohol (isopropanol). The problems with any of these alcohols are antibiotic resistance issues and concerns that the microbiome (the beneficial microorganisms of the skin) may be affected. There doesn't seem to be any bacterial resistance to 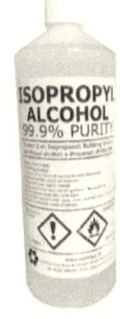 alcohol - so there are no alcohol-resistant bacteria because there are antibiotic-resistant bacteria. The impact of alcohol on the skin on the microbiome is not final. The concern is comparable with antibiotics and their disruptive effects on the intestinal flora of the intestine. In this case, the jury has not yet been decided. But it is advised to be cautious and tends to use disinfectants to a limited extent or not at all so as not to impair the natural flora of the skin. Now let's take a look at obsessive hand disinfection. Alcohol can dry out on the skin and interacts with the lipid barrier - the protective layer of the skin - which provides a barrier and partial immunity to the skin. A report found that healthcare professionals who used an alcohol-based disinfectant did not break down the lipid barrier when the disinfectant also contained a moisturizer. Many disinfectants contain aloe or glycerin, which are considered moisturizers.

Try to exercise caution with constant use of alcohol disinfectants and strongly recommend that if excessive disinfection is required, use a hand cream that contains lipids similar to those found in the skin barrier

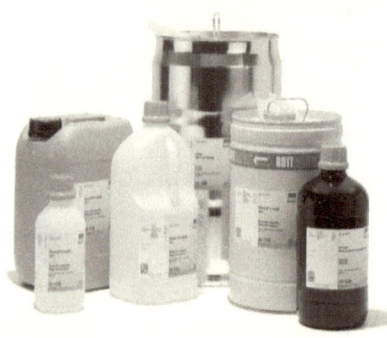

throughout the day. You should also avoid everything with Triclosan. Wash your hands frequently - although this can cause skin irritation that is bigger than an alcohol disinfectant if the soaps are too hard, which is what most of them are. If you need to use an ethanol-based alcohol disinfectant, do so only when needed. Stop being paranoid and germicidal, as this can cause unnecessary stress. The best advice is to spread your immune system and your resistance to pathogens through a healthy diet, nutritional supplements, adequate sleep, stress relief and a few daily drops of essential oil such as diluted in massage oil, MQV, and rub it over your chest and back Knees and feet.

Depending on the active ingredients used, hand sanitizers can be divided into two types: alcohol-based or alcohol-free. Alcohol-based products usually contain

60-95% alcohol, usually in the form of ethanol, isopropanol, or n-propanol. At these concentrations, alcohol quickly denatures proteins and effectively neutralizes certain types of microorganisms. 2,4,6 alcohol-free products are generally based on disinfectants such as benzalkonium chloride (BAC) of antibacterial agents such as triclosan 1,6,7. Disinfectant and antimicrobial activity are immediate and permanent.

USEFULNESS OF ALCOHOL

There are many myths and misunderstandings about hand sanitizers. One of the most popular misunderstandings is that hand sanitizers are practically infallible and can prevent the spread of all contagious diseases, including the common cold or flu. Although a hand sanitizer can kill more than 60 percent of the flu viruses in your hand, most people actually get flu from the air by inhaling the germs. Even if you've used a disinfectant and your hands are clean and germ-free, you can still catch or spread the virus. A hand disinfectant can actually be a more effective preventive mechanism for gastrointestinal diseases than infections such as the common cold or flu. Another myth is that they are not as effective as washing your hands with soap and water to remove germs from your hands. This is not necessarily true. Washing with soap and water works better if your hands are visibly dirty, i.e., if you have dirt in your hands. However, if your hands look clean but are actually littered with germs, an alcohol-based hand disinfectant is a better option because the alcohol kills the germs more effectively. Another myth is that hand disinfectants lead to dry hands. These products contain emollients, chemicals that reduce irritation by protecting and soothing the skin. As catchy as it may seem, an alcohol-based hand disinfectant is less damaging to the skin than soap and water. A hand disinfectant, on the other hand, can moisturize the hands.

You can make a somewhat effective disinfectant at home. While homemade variants can be cheaper, most don't contain the recommended alcohol content of 60 percent. Experts agree that this is the optimal concentration for eliminating germs. Understandably, the best results are achieved with brand names such as Purell or Germ X. However, as long as the product contains 60 percent alcohol, a generic brand works just as well as a premium private label. There is no need to pay higher prices for branded products. If we summarize all the facts about hand disinfectants, we can say with certainty that an alcohol-based disinfectant is the most effective way to kill germs in our hands, but only as long as the product is used sparingly and responsibly. An alcohol-based disinfectant can not only remove more germs than soap and water but also protects the skin if used in moderate amounts. And if an adult supervises it, this product can also be safe for children. While alcohol-based disinfectants have recently been criticized primarily for their high alcohol concentration, experts say that some of these fears are unfounded. Alcohol is in no way absorbed by the skin to justify these fears. Even with excessive use, alcohol intake is harmless at best.

Alcohol can contribute to some disinfectant hazards, but not to a large extent. The argument against alcohol content only persists if the products are used in such a way that they were not intended for use. For example, an alcohol-based hand disinfectant should not be taken, but there have been several cases in which both children and adults have consumed the liquid and have become very ill. Some manufacturers have tried to address public concern about alcohol levels and have started to produce non-alcoholic alternatives as a safer alternative. These products rely on vegetable oils to neutralize germs but have not been as effective as alcohol-based hand disinfectants. When used properly, an alcohol-based hand disinfectant is no more dangerous than an alcohol-free version.

FOAM HAND DISINFECTANT

Hand disinfectants are an integral part of the office and household cleaning products, and foam hand disinfectant is one of the most environmentally-friendly hygiene products. Some of the other products provided under the same category are the Cutan hand disinfectant, the Deb hand disinfectant, and the hand disinfectant gel. As part of hand cleaning solutions, foam disinfectants are characterized by an immediate disinfection effect and are user-friendly. Environmentally friendly hygiene products that not only meet environmental

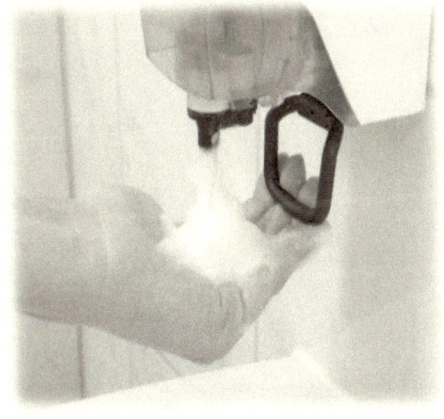

specifications but are also often used to promote the health and hygiene concept. Therefore, they are often used as part of office cleaning products as well as household cleaning products. The Cutan disinfectant is one of the hand disinfectants that are manufactured according to the standards that are specifically required for environmentally-friendly hygiene products. This disinfectant gel belongs to the family of other similar products such as the Deb disinfectant and the foam hand disinfectant. Its credibility involves the fact that it is able to remove 99.99% of bacterial and other harmful microorganisms on the hands within a few seconds after rubbing. A variation on this product is the Cutan foam disinfectant. Since both products are available in packs of 12 pump-top bottles with a capacity of 400 ml each, they are economically suitable for use in washrooms in offices, commercial facilities, and public places.

The starter package for hand disinfection gel dispensers consists of three packs of disinfectant gel and

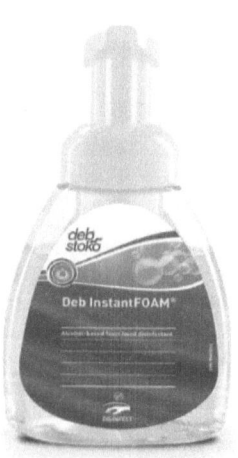

a liter of refills. This product works by providing alcohol hand disinfectants and, together with the Cutan foam disinfectant, is also aptly classified as environmentally friendly hygiene products because it is very effective against MRSA, microbes, germs, and a large number of bacteria that it complies with the antimicrobial standard. The immediate hand disinfectant Gojo Purell belongs to the product range of disinfectants and is intended as an office and home cleaning agent. This hand disinfectant gel is said to perform similar functions to the Cutan hand disinfectant and the Deb hand disinfectant. This foam hand sanitizer can be purchased in a set of twelve bottles to maintain hand hygiene and hand care.

Hand disinfectants and disinfectant wipes are very important in today's heavily polluted environment. They act as protective masks to protect against harmful microbes that cause disease. Regular use of these cleaning solutions is the ideal way to maintain proper personal hygiene. Due to the increasing demand, the market is loaded with a large number of these products. The generous use of hand cleaning disinfectants is one of the most hygienic means to prevent the easy spread of bacteria. These products are said to kill 99.99% of the bacteria on the palm of your hand. The ethyl alcohol contained in these disinfectants is highly effective in destroying the bacteria. They also contain special additives that moisturize your hands and make them soft and refreshed. Hand disinfectants are available in containers with different capacities. For example, they come in 8-ounce pump bottles, 1200 ml bottles, and so on. Popular brands that offer hand sanitizers are Dial, Clorox, Kimberly Clark, and Gojo.

Hand disinfectant dispensers kill bacteria with the active ingredient alcohol. Alcohol makes up between 60 and 90 percent of the disinfectant, and less than 60 percent may not be effective in killing bacteria. The secret is, if alcohol is added to an area that may be filled with bacteria, the particles will be damaged. This only works if the disinfectant is brought into direct contact with the infected area. Hand disinfectants act on the hands but prevent bacteria that can later appear on surfaces. It kills bacteria on contact but is no longer effective afterward. This means that hand disinfectants have to be used all the time, but the high alcohol content can dry out and even irritate the skin. Soap is very different from using a disinfectant. When people wash their hands with soap, bacteria particles are completely removed from the skin. In contrast, disinfectants only neutralize the particles; they are not removed. These particles remain on the skin, but can no longer cause damage. It is best to use both by using the disinfectant after washing your hands. The disinfectant should be rubbed in the hands for about 30 seconds and neutralize a variety of bacteria. It has even been shown to safeguard against MRSA, flu virus bacterium that can be fatal. In order to further promote the many advantages of hand disinfectants, people who use it are also showing a slower development of new bacteria. Everyone has some form of bacteria on their hands at some point. It doesn't prevent all germs as some are in the air, but it's still a great product.

Although hand sanitizer is a wonderful product, it shouldn't be used for everything. For example, if the hands are exposed to blood, they should be washed with soap and water. In addition, it is not a good thing in the foodservice industry because hands get very wet while preparing food and faecal matter on hands after improper hand washing is not properly removed by improper handwashing. When buying a hand disinfectant, check the alcohol content in it. The superior the alcohol concentration, the more effective it is. There are even a variety of scents, and there are even miniature dispensers that can be put in a handbag or travel bag for use. They should be used all year round, but are even better to protect us in the winter months as there are many viruses in circulation.

Given recent concerns about H1N1 and other flu viruses, many people have turned to hand sanitizers to protect their homes and offices. The question is, do they really work, and how safe are they? The first point to note about disinfectants is that they were never intended to be a complete replacement for washing. When a person's hands are dirty, the hand sanitizer alone cannot penetrate all of the dirt and grease required for proper cleaning. Another important point to emphasize is that in order to take advantage of the disinfectant, the individual must use the same discretion as to when washing - that is, the disinfectant must be thoroughly rubbed into all surfaces of the hand to achieve maximum effectiveness. While automatic disinfectant dispensers obviously have the advantage of reducing cross-contamination by not having to touch the device itself, any system is only as good as its weakest link. If taps, garbage container lids, and bathroom door handles are not cleaned thoroughly, the advantage of an automatic dispenser will be nullified. The same applies to kitchen fittings and sinks, which in many cases, actually represent a larger source of bacteria.

Likewise, the type of disinfectant used in a dispenser can greatly affect its effectiveness. Before investing in a non-contact dispenser, always make sure that the disinfectant recommended by the manufacturer contains at least 60% alcohol. In addition to the way disinfectants work, safety must also be taken into account. Since hand disinfectants usually contain ethyl or isopropyl alcohol, discretion may be required when used in children. In some cases, it is known that children, and especially toddlers, drink the liquid or lick their hands after delivery. In some schools, adults need to administer the disinfectant, but even that doesn't prevent children from biting and licking nails (especially if too much is applied or the type of disinfectant does not dry quickly enough to be monitored). A disinfectant with an alcohol content of 90% is more effective, but it also carries an increased risk. Sometimes the attractive packaging, the colour of the disinfectant, and the fragrance are actually an incentive for problems. For this reason, foaming disinfectant formulas have the advantage that they dry quickly. It is also important to know that hand disinfectant should not be used on open wounds. In addition, not much imagination is required to recognize the potential danger of storing flammable alcohol-based products in hot cars or near other heat sources. Despite safety concerns, hand disinfectants, when used properly, can be an effective tool to prevent the spread of viruses. While there is no guarantee that disinfectants will work against all types of germs, overall, they offer one of the best defense mechanisms against the common cold and flu viruses.

DISINFECTANT WIPES

It may not be possible to wash your hands with soap and water on the way. Disinfectant wipes are available. If you are travelling, you can keep some of them in your pockets or bags. Hand disinfectants are available in a

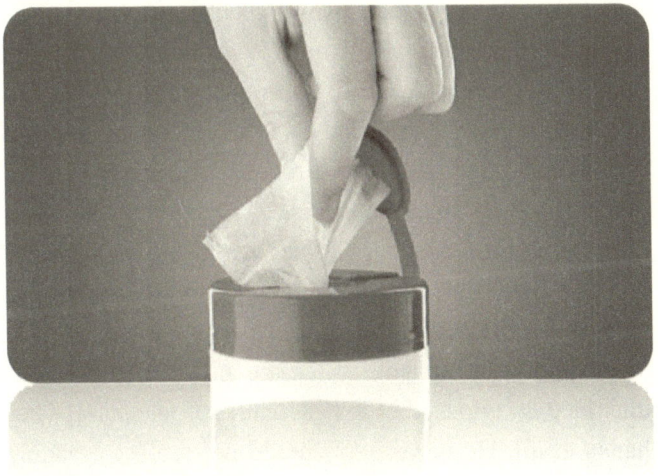

variety of preparations, including gel, foam, and liquid solutions. They are wet wipes that contain a considerable amount of effective cleaning agents. Grease, oil, or any kind of dirt can be effectively removed with disinfectant wipes. The delicate surfaces of these wipes contribute to thorough and effective cleaning. To prevent allergies to the skin, they contain lanolin, aloe skincare products, and mild detergents. These cloth-like disinfectant wipes generally have non-abrasive properties. Superior strength and softness are additional features. If you really care about your personal hygiene and hygiene, it is important to have the required number of hand cleaning and disinfection wipes in stock.

Everyone has some kind of hand disinfectant in his handbag, on his desk, in the car. Children have hand disinfectants in their book bags, teachers hold bottles on their desks and give towels to their students. But how effective are these hand disinfectants, especially the towels? Are hand disinfectant wipes effective? Although disinfectant manufacturers claim that most wipes kill 99.9% of harmful germs and bacteria, it is found that this is not always the case. These are often tested on lifeless objects, not on hands, and in reality, do not kill as many harmful germs. Much of what the disinfectant wipes remove does not even make people really sick. The perfect way to stay healthy is to wash your hands in soap and water. If soap and water are not available, hand disinfectant wipes are better than not cleaning your hands at all. However, you should not replace washing your hands. The amount of hand disinfectant used should also be kept to a minimum. For example, soap and water should be used where available. If not, remove the wipes for use. Some argue that increased use of hand disinfectant wipes and gels increases disease by killing the good bacteria needed to fight germs and disease-causing bacteria. Some believe that the overuse of hand sanitizers will decrease resistance and increase disease.

Many children are now used to washing their hands with hand disinfectants instead of water and soap. This results in them not washing their hands effectively when using water and soap as they are not practicing enough. This, in turn, can lead to increased disease. However, there is a place and time to use hand disinfectant wipes. Sometimes it is simple or practical to wash your hands with soap and water. Maybe a family is sitting in a car, and someone is sneezing, use the towels. Perhaps a salesperson has just shaken hands with a large number of people and cannot find soap or water. Use a cloth. Sometimes people don't have the mobility or the ability to wash their hands all the time. This is a time when wipes can be useful.

THE LAWS OF HAND DISINFECTANTS

Everyone should know by now that hand disinfectants are essential for maintaining health and protecting your immune system from germs. The Centers for Disease Control (CDC) have informed us that the use of a hand sanitizer to remove germs washes hands not only frequently and thoroughly, but also significantly reduces the risk of colds and flu, among other things. Here are the three laws to look for when looking for a good hand sanitizer.

The law of effectiveness: To be viable as a disinfection product, you need a hand disinfectant that WORKS. There are so much products on the market, but the FDA has specifically approved certain substances as antimicrobial agents. One of these substances is ethyl alcohol. In the right amounts, ethyl alcohol can be 99.9% effective against germs. The usual amount is between 62 and 70% by volume. If a hand sanitizer doesn't contain an FDA-approved drug, such as ethyl alcohol, you can't be sure that it will work.

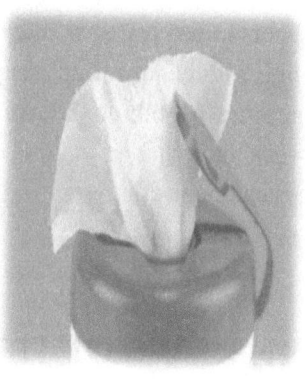

The law of application: Hand disinfection is not something that the majority of people do regularly. The problem is that they should, but most hand sanitizers are painful to apply. You need to pull out a tiny bottle, open the cap, squeeze out the gel in the right amount, and try to spread it on your hands before it slips or evaporates. It's a simple feat for people with more than two hands, but a little complicated for the rest of us. The best application for hand disinfectants is via a spray bottle, which delivers the right amount per spray and is very easy to use with two hands. If you can't easily use the hand sanitizer, why should you be motivated to use it?

The law of moisture: Alcohol is a solvent that extracts natural oils from things it touches, including your skin. When your skin looses its natural oils, it dries out. This can be painful, and yet another reason why people don't want to use hand sanitizers. For this reason, the Moisture Act states that you should receive a hand disinfectant with aloe or essential oils! The alcohol evaporates after rubbing it around to kill germs, and you get a pleasant moisturizing solution that prevents your hands from cracking and pain. Follow these laws, and you will find a great hand sanitizer that is painless! Hand disinfection is one of the best ways not to get sick. So don't be afraid any more - follow the 3 laws for hand disinfectants and protect yourself!

MAKE YOUR OWN HOMEMADE HAND SANITIZER

The cold and flu period is in full swing, and since H1N1 runs everywhere, it's never bad to take a few extra precautions to keep germs at bay. Washing your hands with soap and water always is still the best way to get rid of germs. But after an excursion that exposes you to a lot of germs (like the grocery, gas pump, public bathrooms), killing some of these foreign attackers if you don't have access to a sink and soap is a good idea. There are many, many hand sanitizer products on the market, but you can make your own hand sanitizer at a fraction of the cost. Most of the products you buy are alcohol-based, but while green enthusiasm continues, more natural products made with essential oils find their way onto the market. If you choose an alcohol-based product, make sure that it has an alcohol concentration of at least 60 percent, so that most of the harmful bacteria and viruses are killed. Check these labels on your hand sanitizers, so you know they actually do the job and not just smear the germs. Essential oils have been used to fight disease for thousands of years, and you may already have all the oils in your home that are required to make your own hand sanitizer. By using essential oils with disinfectant, antiseptic, and antiviral properties, you can make a homemade hand disinfectant without alcohol. Cedarwood, lavender, lemon, lemongrass, myrrh, neroli, patchouli, peppermint, rose, sandalwood, tea tree, thyme, and ylang-ylang essential oils all have antiseptic properties. Clove, Niaouli, and pine oils have both a disinfectant and antiseptic properties. Tea tree oil is the strongest of these antiseptics, but should not be used by children or pregnant / breastfeeding women. Adding more tea tree oil to a recipe will make the hand sanitizer more effective, but the smell can be overwhelming. A little drop of essential oils such as basil, rosemary, rose, lavender, lemon, or geranium will brighten and balance it with a nice smell.

Always be careful with basic oils and consult your doctors before using if you suffer from current health conditions. As already mentioned, some oils (such as tea tree, cedar, and hyssop) are not suitable for children or pregnant and lactating women. In the following recipes, you can mix oils to your taste or just use one type of oil. A safe family option for essential oil blends is a combination of lavender and pine. This creates a disinfectant, antiseptic hand disinfectant with a calming effect. Add a little citron or rosemary to enhance and round off the aroma. Aloe vera gel is part of all these recipes and to mention that this means pure aloe vera gel with no colouring, aroma, etc. It is not the same as juice. "100% Aloe Vera Gel" should appear somewhere on the bottle. If not, it's the wrong stuff. If you're finding it difficult to get one of these ingredients in your local stores, try online sources.

However, it is essential to note that antibacterial is not the same as antiviral. Because of some virus, some

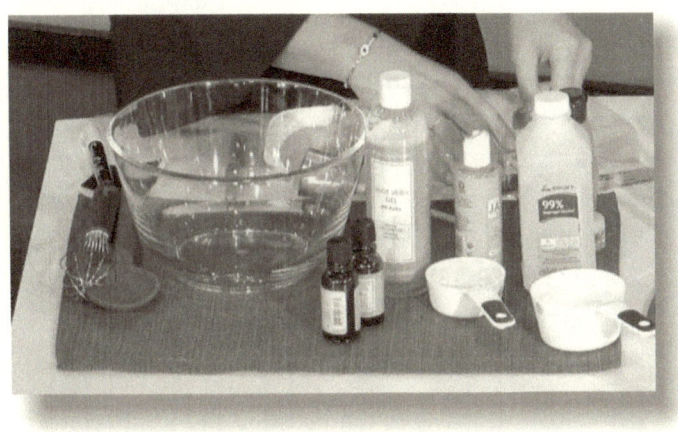

essential oils with antibacterial properties may not be as effective. "They all have antibacterial properties, which is why you need them. To put it bluntly: although you do-it-yourself, disinfectants are not recommended as 100% protection, here is the breakdown if you are trying to do so. Hand disinfectants can be made at home using three main ingredients: isopropyl alcohol (91 percent or more), aloe vera gel, and a few drops of essential oil. Before you put all of these ingredients together, there are a few things you should know. Isopropyl alcohol is the main ingredient of disinfection in this DIY hand disinfection recipe. Use alcohol with an alcohol content of 91 percent or more to make your home disinfectant as effective as possible. Ideally, 99 percent is the best thing you can do, but anything over 91 still works efficiently to kill germs and bacteria.

Here are the homemade recipes for hand disinfectants with and without alcohol. Mixing a batch of hand sanitizer takes just a few minutes, but the question that often arises is what you have at home. You may want to do the mixing in a glass bowl (plastic can take on the aroma of the essential oils and metal can react with the ingredients), but you can also pour the ingredients at once into a bottle if you prefer. In any case, a funnel will be useful. Add ingredients to mixing bowl and shake or stir. Fill the mixture into washed hand sanitizer and other small bottles. Some more fluid recipes may need to be shaken before using to dispense the oil.

Hundreds of diseases can be detected by skin contact today. But we cannot stop ourselves or our children from holding and touching objects found in public places where germs can be found most of the time. So it's not a bad thing to take extra precautions. Wash your hands with soap that is the best way to prevent yourself from germs. But as we all know, it is not very easy. Wherever you go, most importantly, when you are with your family, if you can't get soap and water, it is recommended that you disinfect your hands with a hand sanitizer. There are many types of hand sanitizers you can find on the market. The best are those with an alcohol concentration of 60-80%, as they are very effective at disinfecting and killing bacteria. You can also decide to use a natural oil-based disinfectant with disinfectant properties. Essential oils from cedarwood, cloves, lavender, lemon, pine, tea tree, and ylang-ylang have antiseptic and disinfectant properties. However, tea tree oil is the strongest of these oils because it also contains antiviral, antifungal, and antibacterial properties. Whatever you choose, the disinfectant must contain a moisturizer so that your hands and skin do not dry out. Now, if you want to make sure that the hand sanitizer that you and your family use is used, you can make your own hand sanitizer. You save money and can choose the ingredients to be used personally.

What is social distancing, how can it stop the spread of flu virus - and tips and tricks from making it easier. Alternatively, if you have access to an aloe vera plant, you can cut from the plant and use it for its healing (and disinfecting) properties. It is also vital for the recipe because of its moisturizing properties. It prevents your skin from drying out. Without adding aloe vera to it, the alcohol in this hand disinfection recipe would cause your skin to dry out. When it comes to crucial oils, there are some that you can use as a disinfectant. By far, however, the most recommended essential oil for disinfectants is the tea tree. Tea tree oil has antibacterial properties as well as anti-inflammatory, antifungal, and antiviral properties. While research is limited on which viruses can successfully fight the tea tree essential oil, it is believed to fight off the pathogens associated with acne, staphylococci, micrococci, Enterococcus faecalis, and Pseudomonas aeruginosa. Cinnamon is another recommended vital oil for making hand sanitizers. If you're just looking for a hand sanitizer that smells good, use lemon, orange, peppermint, or lavender. No matter which essential oil you choose, 8-15 drops should do the trick. In support of these three main ingredients, you will likely need a mixing bowl, spoon, measuring cup, and funnel. These things are not necessary, but they definitely make the measuring and cleaning process considerably easier!

NON-ALCOHOLIC HAND DISINFECTANT GEL

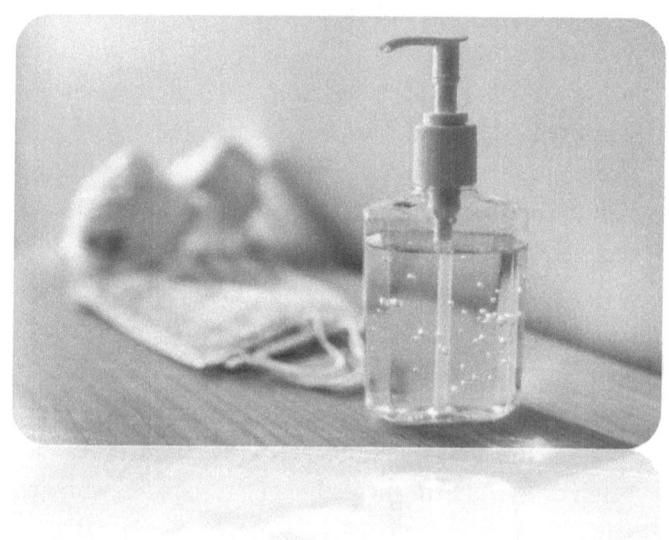

* 1 cup of pure aloe vera gel

* 1/2 cup of vitamin E.

* 1-2 teaspoons of witch hazel (add until the required consistency is achieved)

* 8 drops of essential oils (depending on your preferences)

Mostly alcohol hand disinfectant gel

2 cups of pure aloe vera gel

2 tablespoons of 90% SD40 alcohol (perfumer alcohol if you can get it)

2-3 teaspoons of essential oils

Alcohol-based hand disinfectant

1/4 cup of clear aloe vera gel

1/4 cups of grain alcohol or vodka

10 drops of essential oils

Important things you should know about hand disinfectants

Most people have probably heard that hand disinfectants are effective in killing germs. Yes, that's right, but why is it so effective? Is it better to wash your hands with soap and water or use a hand sanitizer? Hand disinfectants work due to their high alcohol concentration, and alcohol kills most germs and bacteria. Rubbing alcohol on your hands for about 30 seconds will kill off many forms of bacteria and viruses. An interesting statistic is that a person using disinfectants is also likely to experience slower bacterial development.

Everyone has some bacteria on their hands at all times, but hand sanitizers slow down the growth of bacteria when used properly. Research as shown that the use of hand disinfectants and other forms of handwashing in schools significantly reduces the disease rate and leads to better attendance lists. In some cases, an alcohol-based disinfectant can also be more effective than hand washing because it is easier and faster to use. For handwashing to be really effective, you need to use warm water, soap, and foam for about 2 minutes. Most people are too impatient for this, so washing your hands won't completely kill the bacteria on your hands. Hand disinfectants, on the other hand, can be carried in small bottles and only take about 30 seconds to kill germs.

Everyone should know that hand sanitizer is great in many cases, but they are not the best choice for ALL cleaning needs. Hand disinfectants are not effective in the food industry, where hands are often wet during preparation. The hand disinfectant does not remove faeces on the hands after poor hand washing after use in the bathroom. In addition, contact with dirt or body fluids requires thorough hand washing. Hand sanitizers shouldn't replace hand washing in all cases, but it can be a great way to kill germs and bacteria, especially when you're on the go.

Put a small amount (about the size of your thumbnail) on the palm of your hand. Rub it over your entire hand and your nail beds. You would know that if the gel evaporated completely in less than 15 seconds, you would not have used enough. The alcohol content of hand cleaners can be in the form of ethyl alcohol, ethanol, or isopropanol. Regardless of what type of alcohol is listed, its concentration should be between 60 and 95 percent. Less than 60 percent is not enough to be an effective cleaning agent. While alcohol consumption is common, some groups have advocated keeping alcohol-based ones away from children. You could lick the gels off your hands, and this can lead to alcohol poisoning! This homemade disinfectant is suitable for all skin types. However, keep in mind that this is not meant to be a substitute for soap and water. Their use is, at most, a supplementary habit. This cleaner is most effective when used with careful handwashing.

ALL NATURAL HAND SANITIZER

Ingredients:

1/4 cup witch hazel extract

1/4 cup aloe vera gel

1 teaspoon. vegetable glycerin

1 TBSP. Lemon juice or organic apple cider vinegar

10 drops of tea tree oil

Directions:

1. Put all the ingredients in a bottle with a lid and mix.

2. Place a swab on your hands and massage it into your skin.

3. Rinse off with warm water.

One of the gates of the deadly viruses and bacteria is our mouth, and our hand serves as a viaduct. What doctors and health experts say, always wash your hands. The purpose of this event is to tell people to wash their hands as an everyday habit. Nevertheless, not everyone can have clean water and disinfectant soap and wash their hands everywhere. Here are the simple steps to making a bottle of homemade hand sanitizer. When formulating a cheap custom item like a homemade disinfectant, you need:

Half a cup of 99.9% alcohol

The fourth cup of aloe vera gel

Volatile oil

Natural dye

Press the bottle

Method:

Combine all ingredients until everything is thoroughly combined. Simply add a few drops of essential oil and dye to your preferred fragrance and colour. Just get a big bottle and pour the mixture into it. Bring it with you wherever you go to be safe. The intention of this homemade disinfectant to ensure health security outside the home is undeniable.

ESSENTIAL OILS IN HAND DISINFECTANT

The essential oil you choose not only gives your hand disinfectant fragrances but also protects you from germs. If you are using antimicrobial oils, use only a drop or two as these oils are very strong and can irritate your skin. Other oils like lavender or chamomile can soothe your skin. Tea tree oil is antimicrobial. A few drops can be added to the recipe, but it is important to note that many people are very sensitive to this oil, even if it is diluted. What you will need. Equipment / tools:

Bowl and spoon

Funnel

Bottle with a pump dispenser

Materials:

2/3 cup of 99 percent alcohol (isopropyl alcohol) or ethanol

1/3 cup aloe vera gel

8 to 10 drops of basic oil, optional

Steps to do Make hand sanitizer:

1. Once you gather your ingredients. Make sure you have your cleansing alcohol, aloe vera gel, and optional essential oils ready and measured.

2. Mix ingredients. Add all the ingredients together in your bowl and mix thoroughly with a spoon.

3. Pour into your bottle. When you are using the funnel, carefully pour your DIY hand sanitizer into the bottle of your choice, screw the lid of your bottle on, and start using it.

Substitutions:

The main component of the hand disinfectant is alcohol, so it is possible to replace the aloe vera gel. The purpose of aloe gel is to protect the hands from the dehydration effects of alcohol. Basically, it's a humectant. This means that it helps trap moisture. Other humectants that could be used in place of aloe include glycerin or hand lotion. However, it is still important to keep the alcohol in the final product at least 60%. If you don't find alcohol, it's best to wash your hands with soap and water instead of trying a homemade hand sanitizer recipe.

Work with 70% alcohol - Alcohol and ethanol from a store are usually either 90-99% alcohol or 70% alcohol. You can use 70% of alcohol to disinfect your hands, but you can add very little (possibly a few drops of essential oil or jojoba oil to improve the smell or texture). By mixing 70% alcohol with other ingredients, the alcohol is diluted so that the alcohol content recommended by the CDC can easily fall below 60%.

Protect your hands - Alcohol dries skin and removes protective oils. Use a hand sanitizer (or hand wash) with a good lotion to keep the skin in shape. Damaged skin has small cracks that trap bacteria and viruses and make removal difficult. If your skin is sensitive, try to keep the amount of alcohol in your hand disinfectant around 60-70% as in this recipe. Higher concentrations can cause irritation.

HAND WASHING AND HAND DISINFECTANT

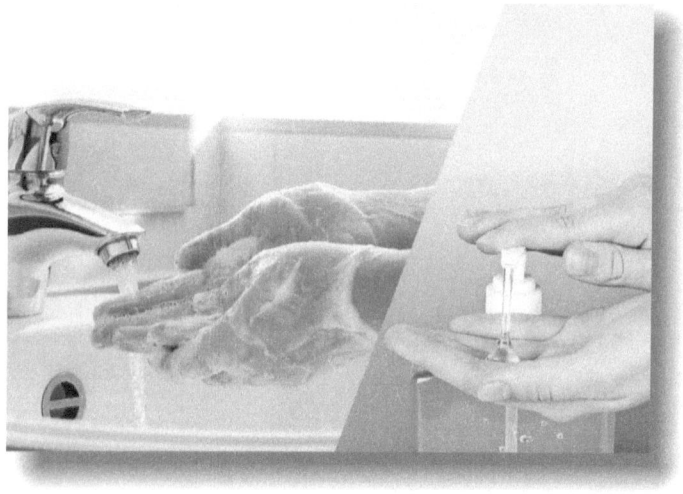

It may surprise you that 80% of all infections are transmitted by hand. Simple good hygiene can prevent the spread of germs and the transmission of bacteria and viruses that can cause illness. This is especially important during the cold and flu season and on special holidays, which are the crucial times of the year, to keep germs out. Who wants to get sick in these special times?

Here's what you need to know. There are basically two options.

Old-fashioned hand washing comes first. You have to wash your hands properly and often. Moisten your hands with warm, running water, apply soap, lather and rub it with soap quickly for at least 15 seconds. It is important to clean between your fingers, under your fingernails, the back of your hand, and even your wrists. You should rinse your hands well and dry them with a clean towel or paper towel. Use a toilet roll to turn off the taps and open the door when you leave as both are germ carriers. When

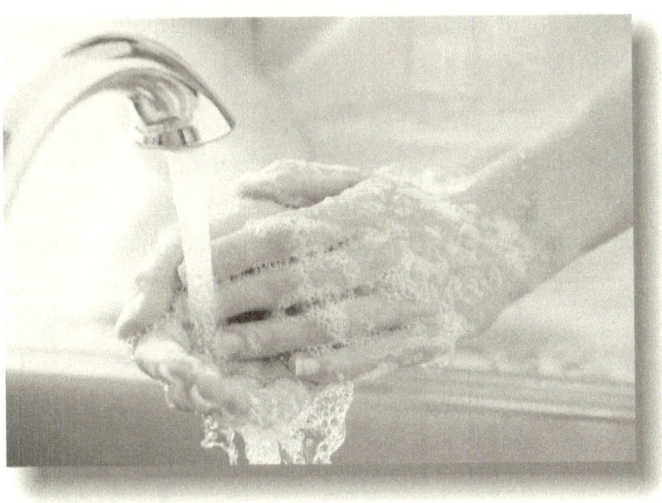

should you wash your hands? You'd think it was a no-brainer, but apparently, there are a lot of people out there who don't wash when they should.

Here are guidelines to help you know when you need to wash your hands: before and after preparing your food, before and after eating, after sneezing or coughing, nasal brushing, using a public washroom, dealing with pets, changing diapers, washing and the remote control, computer keyboard and so on. Washing hands is easy and effectively prevents the spread of germs. Nevertheless, life is busy, and access to water and soap is not always possible. An alternative to washing hands is to use a hand disinfectant. There are non-alcoholic hand disinfectants. Both kill 99.9% of the bacteria within 15 seconds, but alcohol-free hand sanitizers are easy, non-toxic, non-flammable, and safe for the whole family. Alcohol-based disinfectants dry your skin and cause small cracks and a fissures-the the perfect place to hide bad, disease-causing bacteria!

An alcohol-free hand disinfectant contains germicidal benzalkonium chloride and feels better on your skin than alcohol-based disinfectants. It leaves no sticky residue and makes your skin soft, moisturized, and, above all, germ-free. A hand disinfectant is also effective in killing germs that can cause disease, including Norwalk virus, SARS, avian, salmonella, E. coli, and more. Another good thing about hand sanitizers is that you can take them with you when you're on the go and when handwashing may not be possible. Many come in mini sprays that fit comfortably in your pocket, wallet, purse, backpack, computer bag, or briefcase. Some offer large sizes for your home that your whole family can use. And if you are travelling for business or pleasure, the mini sprays are excellent companions. You can take them with you, whether you are sightseeing or relaxing in the sun on a beautiful beach.

Using a hand sanitizer is easy. Simply apply a thumbnail to the palm of your hand, just enough to make your skin feel wet. Rub it in your hands until it's dry. Within 15 seconds, it killed 99.9% of the germs that caused the disease. The main goal is to stay healthy, and both hand washing and hand sanitizer are great ways to prevent the spread of disease-causing germs. Prevention is invaluable.

HOW DOES HAND DISINFECTANT WORK?

You have probably heard that hand disinfectants are effective hand cleaners that kill germs and bacteria, but have you ever wondered how a simple alcohol-based hand disinfectant could be as effective as thorough hand soap and water wash? Hand soap and water lift the germs from our skin and rinse them off, while hand disinfectants only kill the germs on contact. This is quite remarkable, and the question is, how? Hand disinfectants consist of ethyl alcohol, inactive additives such as water, other alcohols, and fragrances. Ethyl alcohol is the active ingredient and is said to kill germs. An important note about ethyl alcohol is that it is only effective if the alcohol concentration is between 60 and 95%. Less than 60% is not enough to kill germs and is pointless to use.

Many experts have pointed out that it is very important to read the labels on the hand sanitizers to ensure that you are getting a quality product with sufficient alcohol levels. There are two general types of alcohol: ethyl alcohol and isopropyl alcohol. Both types kill bacteria sufficiently but are not as effective on viruses. When the alcohol evaporates, it sucks out the inside of bacteria and viruses and kills them. However, the bacteria or viruses will only be dead once all of the alcohol has evaporated. One thing to note is that isopropyl alcohol takes about 10 minutes on the surface of the skin to kill bacteria, which gives ethyl alcohol an advantage over isopropyl alcohol.

When applying the hand sanitizer, be sure to rub every part of the skin thoroughly on your hands as this will kill the germs. Hand disinfectants do not get through body fluids, dirt, blood, or other dirt to kill germs. These things need to be washed off before using a hand sanitizer. The alcohol in the hand disinfectant also has a drying effect. Therefore, it is a very nice idea to use some kind of hand or body lotion after using the hand sanitizer.

Let's say you have just eaten your hamburger and have access to a hand sanitizer, water, and soap. Which one should you choose? Our parents have been telling us about the importance of washing hands for years, but today people are asking whether hand disinfectants are more effective at killing germs than our old friend soap and water. The answer is yes. Nowadays, most hand disinfectants use ethyl alcohol or isopropyl alcohol (or a mixture thereof) as an active ingredient to kill 99.99% of the germs on the hands. The active ingredient ethyl alcohol or isopropyl alcohol has the ability to immediately break down the cell walls of the germs and let them perish. However, to kill 99.99% of the germs, a hand sanitizer must contain between 60% and 90% alcohol. Soap is actually not a germicide or antiseptic. There are dead cells, dried sweat, various germs on your hands, and dust. The speciality of soap is its ability to get rid of it mechanically. If you only wash your hands with water, the oil layer on your hands prevents the water from reacting with the skin and minimizes hygiene. Normal soaps are made up of different types. Molecules are hydrophilic (water-binding), and the other is hydrophobic (water-repellent). When you rub your hands with soap and water, soap molecules break down the oil layer, while water washes away the germs and dirt. In the end, however, the percentage of germs killed by the combination of soap and water will be less than 99.99%.

Make it a habit to use hand disinfectants. Do you remember this old nursery rhyme that says: "Clean little hands are easy to see!"? Well, our hands are no longer small, but they always have to be clean! We all know how important it is to wash our hands properly, but when soap and water are not available, we turn to our reliable hand sanitizer to get the job done. Hand disinfectants are gels that contain alcohol that is said to kill bacteria and viruses. Because alcohol can cause dryness, most brands contain moisturizers to minimize dryness and irritation to the skin. Several research studies have shown that the use of hand cleaners in families reduces the risk of spreading gastrointestinal and respiratory infections. It is, therefore, good to always have one in your handbag.

HANDWASHING TECHNIQUES TO PROTECT YOUR CHILD FROM FLU AND OTHER VIRUSES

Children are their own worst enemies when it comes to the flu season. Having clean hands is the best deterrent. Unfortunately, children and clean hands don't go well together! Children (of all ages) touch everything in sight.

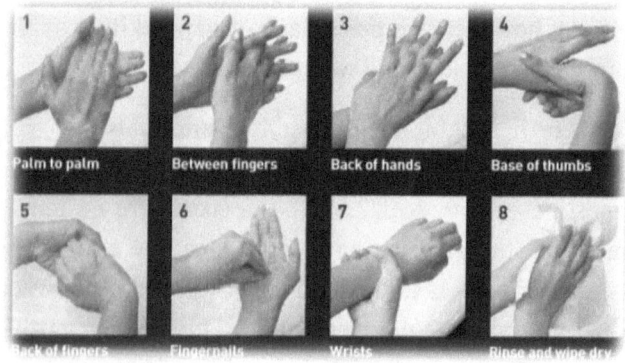

The younger they are, the easier they have access to the most disgusting and germ-infested surfaces, e.g., under tables, shoes, trash cans, and this is worst for our little crawlers. When touching these dirty surfaces is not rough enough. The next thing you do is take a handful of fingers and put them in your mouth! So our children get sick all the time. The germs from your fingers go either into your mouth or into your eyes, where the virus can get into your body. If your child is trained in the potty, they can most likely wash their own hands, but the problem is that they are often too distracted even to consider washing their hands. They don't care, they don't understand it and most of all they don't want to stop playing.

We want to give our children the habit of washing their hands. The best way to create a habit for children is to make them a fun activity. How is washing hands fun? Here are guides to assist you in getting started:

- Sweets work! Tell your child that every time they wash their hands, they get a piece of their favourite candy. Make it a double hit by making the "candy" out of these little kid vitamins (flint or these fun gums work well).

- For the older ones. Make it a competition and give the winner a prize (works well with multiple children). Tell your children every time they wash their hands that they get the point. Whoever reaches the specified points first will receive a prize (favourite food, toys from the dollar store, sweets). If they are really active and playing, it is good once or twice an hour, and at the end of each day, the points are counted.

- If your child is old enough, playfully teach them germs. One method I've heard is to get some baby powder and put it on your children's hands. Tell them to walk around and touch a few things (MESSY! You tell yourself. Of course! This will help make the lesson unforgettable. Relax, it washes off.) Tell your child after some time to look around and see everything that knows!

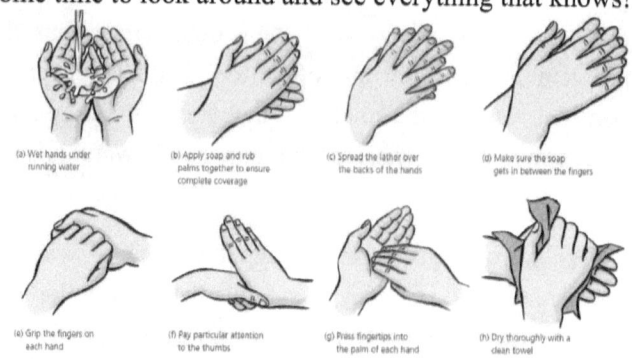

(a) Wet hands under running water
(b) Apply soap and rub palms together to ensure complete coverage
(c) Spread the lather over the backs of the hands
(d) Make sure the soap gets in between the fingers
(e) Grip the fingers on each hand
(f) Pay particular attention to the thumbs
(g) Press fingertips into the palm of each hand
(h) Dry thoroughly with a clean towel

So show them that our germs get on everything!

-To make the actual handwashing process more entertaining. Try the new foam soap that you can get in any store. Children LOVE making the foam. Sometimes they stand there for a long time and just play with the soap in the sink. What a great place to play!

-To make it really fun, get a "Soapy Automatic Soap Dispenser." This works well for mothers and children. "Soapy" has a sensor that releases a pre-measured amount of soap when activated. This often results in the children staying at the sink to wash their hands too. It also makes it a fun time instead of the boredom that it usually is.

"Soapy" also helps mothers out there with babies. Tired of holding your baby and squeezing the soap dispenser? With an automatic soap dispenser, simply put your baby's hand under the dispenser, and it's done, no more balancing! What a great idea. Whatever method you develop, help your children by developing good hygiene practices. Clean hands are important to protect your little ones from the dreaded flu and other viruses. "

• Hand disinfectants are convenient, portable, easy to use, and not time-consuming.

• Several studies have shown that families using hand sanitizers reduce the risk of the spread of gastrointestinal and respiratory infections.

• Commercially manufactured hand disinfectants contain ingredients that prevent skin dryness. Using these products can result in less dryness and skin irritation than washing your hands.

• Studies show that adding hand disinfectants to classrooms can reduce student absenteeism by 20 percent. In addition, many children think that instant hand disinfectants are fun.

Restrictions:

• Not all hand disinfectants are manufactured in the same way. Check the bottle for active ingredients. The alcohol content can be in the form of ethyl alcohol, ethanol, or isopropanol. All of these are acceptable forms of alcohol. Make sure that regardless of the type of alcohol, the concentration is between 60 and 95 percent. The alcohol content of less than 60 percent is not enough to be effective.

• Alcohol does not cut through dirt. Dirt, blood, and dirt must first be wiped or washed off if the alcohol is to be effective in the disinfectant. In such cases, it is recommended to wash your hands with soap and water.

• Hand disinfectants are not cleaning agents and are not intended to replace water and soap, but rather as a supplementary habit. Disinfectants are most effective when used in conjunction with careful handwashing.

The use of hand disinfectants is a habit that can help all of us to be less exposed to germs and therefore reduce the risk of illness. Whether you're in the playground, using someone else's computer, or visiting a friend in the hospital, take your time to rub your hands. It is an easy step towards a healthy winter season.

HOW TO IDENTIFY WHICH HAND WASHING METHOD TO USE

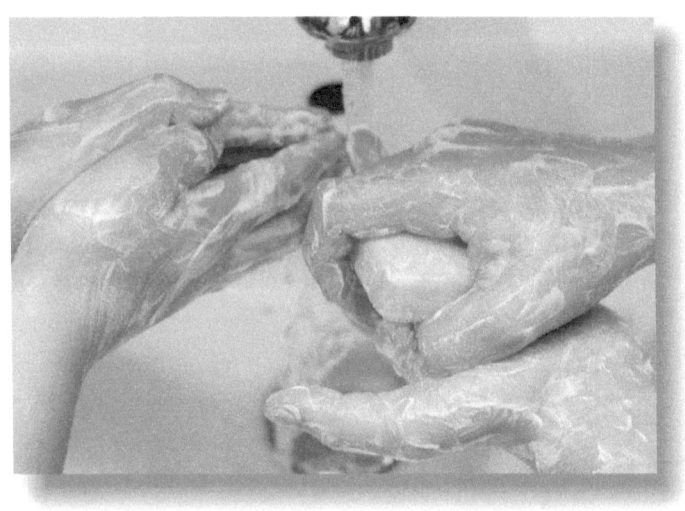

The recommendations for handwashing and hand disinfection for different groups of people may vary depending on their professional functions and personal health requirements. Research has shown that hand disinfectants can only be as effective as washing hands in certain situations. The type of floor that can be present on the hands can significantly change the effectiveness of hand disinfectants. It is significant to wash your hands first with soap and water, like dirt, food, and other items on your hands can reduce the effect of alcohol on the disinfectant. "Recommendation of alcohol-based gels as a suitable replacement for hand washing for healthcare professionals." Many healthcare workers routinely need to wash their hands several times an hour while moving between patients. It has been shown that the use of alcohol gels by staff has a positive impact on hand cleaning due to the time saved compared to conventional hand washing methods. However, only the guidelines for hospitals and clinics apply. These are not suitable for people and do NOT apply to people who work in the catering trade or public. The main reason is that the types and levels of the soil on the hands are very different between these different settings. In hospitality, faeces and enteric viruses such as the norovirus are a bigger problem. Food workers often have wet hands that are contaminated with foods high in protein or fat. Food proteins and fats can reduce the effectiveness of an alcohol gel. Therefore, soap, rubbing, and running water still remain the most effective way to remove the types of pathogens kers might encounter. The FDA rules and regulations of the Model Food Code stipulate that food workers may use hand disinfectants in addition, but not instead of proper handwashing. Since hand disinfectants are considered a food additive, only products from the FDA can be used. Hand washing guidelines for healthcare professionals should not be confused with recommendations for workers or the general public in the food industry. Washing hands with soap and water are sufficient for everyone and is still a must. For the general public at home, soap and water are adequate for most consumer purposes. The additional precaution to use an alcohol gel or an antibacterial soap only in situations such as

1. Physical contact with people at high risk of infection (newborns, very elderly people, immunosuppressed people, etc.)

2. Direct physical contact with people with upper respiratory tract infections, skin infections, or diarrhea; and

3. Working in environments where infectious diseases are common, e.g., in the preparation of food or in crowded living areas (daycare centers, preschools, prisons, or nursing homes).

How different soaps work:

Chemically speaking, "soaps" are potassium salts of fatty acids or water-soluble sodium that have extraordinary properties as surfactants. Antimicrobial soaps contain an antiseptic in addition to mechanical removal to reduce the number of microbes. Triclosan is the most commonly used chemical component in antibacterial soaps. However, a significant key factor for the effectiveness of these soaps is the length of time they stay on the skin and the concentration of the products.

Companies have not released information about which combination of triclosan concentrations and wash times is most effective. Therefore, it is difficult to know which brands work best. Chloroxylenol is another antimicrobial compound found in some antibacterial soaps. There is concern that the use of antimicrobial soaps can lead to bacterial resistance. While this remains theoretically possible, research has so far found no evidence that this is happening.

Like other consumer goods, high price soap may not be the best quality. If you know the different products and their ingredients, you can choose the right product for the cleaning job and at the right price. Most brands also include a moisturizer to minimize skin irritation. Alcohol works instantly and effectively to kill bacteria and most viruses. The antimicrobial activity of alcohol is its ability to alter microbial proteins. Proteins and fats on dirty hands reduce the effectiveness of alcohol as a disinfectant. Alcohol solutions with 60-95% alcohol are the most effective. Higher concentrations are less useful because proteins cannot be easily denatured without water.

Alcohol gels remove the outer layer of oil on the skin and thus destroy all "temporary" micro-organisms that are present on the surface of the hands. After use, the regrowth of bacteria on the skin usually occurs slowly, which effectively prevents "residual" microflora, which is located in the deeper layers of the skin, from reaching the surface. In other to make it more effective, a drop of a cent-sized alcohol gel should be rubbed into your hands for 30 seconds. If your hands are dry after just 10-15 seconds, you probably haven't used enough disinfectant. Hand sanitizers should be used primarily only as a result of conventional soap and water hand washing, except in conditions where soap and water are not available. In these cases, using alcohol gel is undoubtedly better than nothing.

HOW TO USE HAND SANITIZER

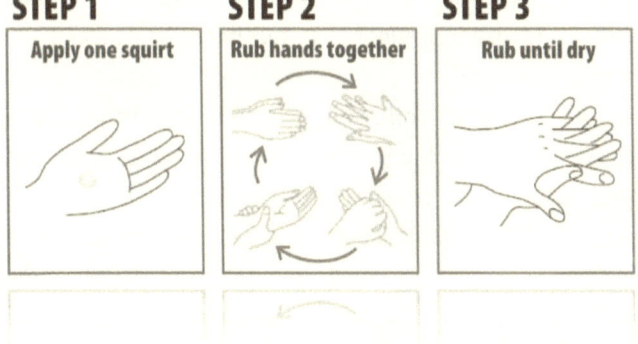

STEP 1 — Apply one squirt

STEP 2 — Rub hands together

STEP 3 — Rub until dry

Two things to keep in mind when using a hand sanitizer are that you need to rub your skin until your hands are dry. But if your hands are greasy or dirty, you should first wash with soap and water. From this perspective, here are some tips for using hand sanitizers effectively. Spray or apply the disinfectant on the palm of your hand. Rub your hands together thoroughly. Be sure to cover the entire surface of your hands and fingers. Continue rubbing for 30-60 seconds or until your hands are dry. It can take a minimum of 60 seconds, and sometimes even longer, for the hand sanitizer to kill most bacteria.

Effectiveness

Before you bother to make the hand sanitizer at home, it is perfectly understandable that you want to know if it is effective. And especially if it is effective against flu virus. The effectiveness of the hand disinfectant depends on several factors, including the way in which the product is used (e.g., the amount used, duration of exposure, frequency of use) and whether the specific infectious agents that are present on the person's hands for the active ingredient is susceptible to the product. In general, alcohol-based hand disinfectants, if rubbed thoroughly over the surface of fingers and hands for 30 seconds, followed by full air drying, can effectively reduce the populations of bacteria, fungi and fungi enveloped viruses (e.g., Influenza A viruses). Similar effects have been reported for certain non-alcoholic formulations such as SAB hand disinfectants (surfactant, and allantoin). However, most hand disinfectants are relatively ineffective against bacterial spores, non-enveloped viruses (e.g., norovirus), and encrypted parasites (e.g., Giardia). They also do not completely cleanse or disinfect the skin if the hands are noticeably dirty before use.

Despite the different efficacy, hand disinfectants can help control the transmission of infectious diseases, especially in environments where washing hands is poor. For example, in primary school children, the inclusion of an alcohol-based or an alcohol-free hand disinfectant in hand hygiene programs in the classroom has been associated with a reduction in absenteeism related to infectious diseases. Also, in the workplace, the use of alcohol-based hand disinfectants has been associated with a decrease in disease episodes and Days of sickness linked. Improved access to alcohol-based hand disinfectants has been linked to general improvements in hand hygiene in hospitals and health clinics.

MYTHS ABOUT HAND DISINFECTANT DISPENSERS

The day does not pass without touching bacteria and harmful bacteria. Germs are everywhere, and germs are inevitable. Frequent contact with everyday objects contributes to the spread of germs. Door handles, computer keyboards, and flat surfaces are just a few of the most popular places where germs can be found. But what can you do to ward off harmful bacteria and germs? Many have turned to hand disinfectants. Hand disinfectants are a great solution to ward off germs. The key to avoiding germs is simply not touching anything you don't need to. Regardless of whether you use a public toilet and use non-contact toilet technology or simply use a standalone hand disinfectant dispenser, not touching devices can reduce the risk of contact with germs. In addition to the hands-free dispenser, many have to choose the gel or foam. Some selected donors actually offer you the options of what you want to see as a donor. This is the choice of a growing number of organizations. You should also be on the lookout for those that are drip-resistant and comply with CDC, APIC, and OSHA standards. This type of dispenser is of the highest quality and meets all sanitary requirements.

Hand disinfectant dispensers generate drug-resistant mutant bacteria. That is wrong. Simply put, alcohol, the main ingredient in hand disinfectant dispensers, kills germs. There is no evidence to support the theory that germs mutate to replace the effects of hand disinfectants. In fact, it has been shown that alcohol-based hand disinfectants even kill multi-resistant pathogens. The best way to be sure that a donor is the right hygiene solution for you is to do a little research. There is a huge amount of research and chemistry that goes into the composition of hand sanitizers. The goal is to protect you by killing the germs that are so easy to come into contact with every day. Focus on your surroundings and make a conservative effort to only touch things in public places that you need to touch. It is also significant to remember that you should wash your hands frequently throughout the day and that you should not touch your eyes, nose, or mouth during the day.

Use hand disinfectant to fight germs - keep employees healthy at work, at home, and on the go. The use of immediate hand disinfectants to fight germs is one of the most basic things in the fight against Flu, colds, and other diseases. There has been a lot of talk about germ-borne diseases lately, especially given the widespread outbreaks of H1N1 swine flu. Hand sanitizers, such as those made by Gojo Industries as part of their Purell hand sanitizers, are a convenient and inexpensive way to combat the spread of such diseases. Where soap and water are not available, hand sanitizers are the next best way to fight bacteria. You can place them in common cars, hallways, offices, bedrooms, and entrances. Shops can place a wall unit near frequently used items such as shopping carts and next to cash registers. Buildings with high concentrations of children and babies are good buildings for the use of hand disinfectants. Curbing germ transmission and spreading disease is significant, especially when young people are involved. Statistics show that the use of hand disinfectants to combat germs at work can significantly reduce employee absenteeism and sick leave. Work performance should also be improved as healthy workers are more alert and work better. Instant hand sanitizers do not require water, and most other hand sanitizers such as towels are also independent of water sources. This is very useful in cases where employees travel and meet large numbers of people.

Shaking hands and using common objects such as telephones, computer keyboards, and input handles can easily spread germs in the office. Take preventive measures and keep bottles of hand sanitizer accessible to everyone at every desk or in a public area. If these types of products are readily available, this should lead to more frequent use. Instructions to employees are also a way to get them to use hand sanitizers regularly. You can buy large industrial quantities, dispensers, or small desktop and personal sizes of hand sanitizers. It is important that the products are available so that they can be used. Also, make sure everyone knows that instant hand sanitizers kill 99.9% of germs and that they are made from materials that soften and moisturize the skin. Using hand disinfectants outside of work is as important as using them at work to ensure employee health. For example, you can give employees the ability to add supplies to their business order that they can use at home for their own deliveries. You should also encourage travelling salespeople to carry hand sanitizers with them and in their vehicles. This improves their chances of avoiding illnesses such as colds and Flu, which cost them money because they are unemployed due to illness. Maintaining a clean and healthy office, benefits everyone, especially the company. It is equally important to keep employees healthy at home and on the go to slow the spread of disease at work. Healthy employees are present at work and tend to do better work.

Some commercially available hand disinfectants contain ingredients that are as scary as the germs they protect you from. So why not make your own hand disinfectant from the ingredients you have selected? This is an excellent project for children and adults as the project can be expanded to include a discussion about hygiene and disinfection. You save money, protect yourself from germs and can adjust the scent of the hand disinfectant so that it does not smell of medication. The active ingredient in this hand disinfectant recipe is the alcohol, which must contain at least 60% of the product in order to be an effective disinfectant. The recipe calls for 99% isopropyl alcohol (cleaning alcohol) or ethanol (grain alcohol, most commonly available from 90% to 95%). Please do not use other types of alcohol (e.g., methanol, butanol) as they are toxic. If you use a product that contains a lower percentage of alcohol (e.g., 70% alcohol), you will need to strengthen the amount of alcohol in the recipe. Otherwise, it will not be as effective.

THE WORLD HEALTH ORGANIZATION'S RECIPE GUIDE

Required materials (small series production)

REAGENTS FOR FORMULATION 1:

- Ethanol 96%

- Hydrogen peroxide 3%

- Glycerin 98%

- Sterile distilled or boiled cold water

REAGENTS FOR FORMULATION 2:

- Isopropyl alcohol 99.8%

- Hydrogen peroxide 3%

- Glycerin 98%

- Sterile distilled or boiled cold water

- 10-liter glass or plastic bottles with a screw cap

- 50-liter plastic tanks (preferably made of polypropylene or high-density polyethylene, translucent to see the liquid level)

• 80-100 liter stainless steel tank (for mixing without overflow)

• Mixing paddles made of wood, plastic or metal

• Measuring cylinder and measuring cup

• Funnel made of plastic or metal

• 100 ml plastic bottles with leak-proof lid

• 500 ml glass or plastic bottles with a screw cap

• An alcoholmeter: the temperature scale is at the bottom, and the ethanol concentration (percentage v / v) is at the top.

NOTE

Glycerin: Used as a humectant, but other emollients can be used for skincare provided they are cheap, widely used, and miscible with water and alcohol and do not add toxicity or promote allergies.

• Hydrogen peroxide: employed to inactivate contaminating bacterial spores in solution and is not an active ingredient in hand disinfection.

• Any further addition to both formulations should be clearly labeled and should not be toxic if accidentally ingested.

• A dye can be added to differentiate it from other liquids but should not contribute to toxicity, promote allergies, or impair antimicrobial properties. Perfume and dye additions are not recommended due to the risk of allergic reactions.

METHOD: 10 LITER PREPARATIONS

These can be made in 10-liter glass or plastic bottles with screw caps. Recommended product quantities:

FORMULATION 1:

- Ethanol 96%: 8333 ml

- Hydrogen peroxide 3%: 417 ml

- Glycerin 98%: 145 ml

FORMULATION 2:

- Isopropyl alcohol 99.8%: 7515 ml

- Hydrogen peroxide 3%: 417 ml

- Glycerin 98%: 145 ml

Step by step preparation:

1. Pour the formula alcohol to be used into a large bottle or tank up to the tick mark.

2. Hydrogen peroxide is added with the measuring cylinder

3. Glycerin is added with a measuring cylinder. Since glycerin is very viscous and sticks to the wall of the meas uring cylind er, it should be rinsed with sterile distilled or cold-boiled water and then emptied into the bottle/tank.

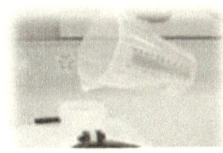

4. The bottle/tank is then filled to the 10-liter mark with sterile distilled or cold boiled water.

5. The lid or screw cap is placed on the tank/bottle as soon as possible after preparation to prevent evaporation.

6. The solution is mixed by agitating gently or with a paddle.

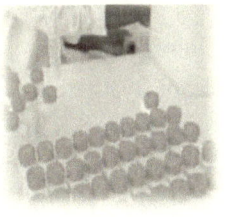

7. Immediately divide the solution into its final container

(e.g., 500 or 100 ml plastic bottles) and quarantine the bottles for 72 hours before use. This enables the destruction of spores in the alcohol or in the new / reused bottles.

End products

FORMULATION 1

Final concentrations:

Ethanol 80% (v / v),

Glycerol 1.45% (v / v),

• Hydrogen peroxide

0.125% (v / v)

FORMULATION 2

Final concentrations:

Isopropyl alcohol 75% (v / v),

Glycerol 1.45% (v / v),

• Hydrogen peroxide

0.125% (v / v)

Quality control

Based on the available knowledge on efficacy, tolerability, and cost-effectiveness, the WHO recommends the use of an alcohol-based hand massage for routine hand antisepsis in most clinical situations. Healthcare facilities currently using commercially available hand rubs, liquid soaps, and skincare products sold in disposable containers should continue this practice provided the hand rubs meet recognized microbicidal effectiveness standards (ASTM or EN standards) and are well approved by the EU / tolerates healthcare workers. It is clear that these products should be considered acceptable, even if their content differs. 1. The pre-production analysis should be performed every time no certificate of analysis is available to ensure the titration of alcohol (i.e., domestic production). Check the alcohol concentration with an alcohol meter and adjust the volume required in the formulation to obtain the final recommended concentration.

2. When employing ethanol or isopropanol solution, post-production analysis is essential. Use the alcohol meter to control the alcohol concentration of the end-use solution. The accepted limits should be set at ± 5% of the target concentration (75% –85% for ethanol).

3. The alcohol meter shown in this information brochure is intended for use with ethanol. When used to control an isopropanol solution, a 75% solution shows 77% (± 1%) on the scale at 25 ° C.

Labeling should comply with national guidelines and include:

- Name of the organization

- Handrub formulation recommended by the WHO

- For external use only

- Avoid contact with the eyes

- Keep away from children

- Date of production and batch number

• Use: Apply a palm of alcohol on a hand base and cover all surfaces of the hands. Rub your hands dry

• Composition: ethanol or isopropanol, glycerin, and hydrogen peroxide

• Flammable: Keep away from flames and heat

Production and storage facilities:

• Ideally, production and storage facilities should be air-conditioned or cool rooms. No open fire or smoking is permitted in these areas.

• Handrub formulations recommended by the WHO should not be produced in quantities of more than 50 liters on-site or in central pharmacies without special air conditioning and ventilation.

• Since undiluted ethanol is easily flammable and can ignite at temperatures of only 10 ° C, production plants should dilute it directly to the above concentration. Flashpoints for ethanol 80% (v / v) and isopropyl alcohol 75% (v / v) are 17.5 ° C and 19 ° C, respectively.

• The national safety guidelines and local legal requirements must be observed when storing the ingredients and the end product.

SAFETY AND COST INFORMATION

The case for alcohol-based hand rubs in healthcare. Currently, alcohol-based hand rubs are the only known way to quickly and effectively inactivate a variety of potentially harmful micro-organisms on the hands. The WHO recommends alcohol-based hand rubs based on the following factors:

1. Evidence-based, intrinsic benefits of a broad-spectrum, fast-acting, microbicidal activity with minimal risk of creating antimicrobial resistance;

2. Suitability for use in resource-restricted or remote areas with inaccessibility to sinks or other hand hygiene facilities (including clean water, towels, etc.);

3. Ability to improve hand hygiene compliance by making the process faster, more convenient, and instantly accessible at the place of patient care;

4. Economic benefits by reducing annual hand hygiene costs, which represent approximately 1% of the additional costs of healthcare-related infections

5. Minimizing the risks of adverse events due to increased security with better acceptance and tolerance than with other products.

Of those of the formulations recommended by the WHO described in this document. The WHO recommends producing the following formulations locally as an alternative if suitable commercial products are either unavailable or too expensive. To help countries and health care facilities change systems and introduce alcohol-based hand rubs, WHO has formulated local formulations. Logistical, economic, security, cultural, and religious factors were carefully examined by the WHO before such formulations were recommended for worldwide use. It is the consensus position of a WHO expert group that hand rub formulations recommended by the WHO can be used both for hygienic hand antisepsis and for preoperative hand preparation.

HYGIENIC HAND RUB

The microbicidal effects of the two formulations recommended by the WHO have been tested by WHO reference laboratories in accordance with the EN standards (EN 1500). It was found that their activity corresponds to the reference substance (isopropanol 60% v / v) for the hygienic hand antisepsis. Both hand-rub formulations recommended by the WHO has been tested by two independent reference laboratories in different European countries in order to assess their suitability for preoperative hand preparation in accordance with the European standard EN 12791. However, although the formulation has not passed the test in both laboratories and formulation II in only one of them, the expert group believes that the microbicidal activity of surgical antisepsis is still a subject for research because of the lack of epidemiological data There is no indication that the effectiveness of n-propanol (propan-1-ol) 60% v / v as a reference in EN 12791 finds a clinical correlate. It is the consensus position of a WHO expert group that the choice of n-propanol as reference alcohol for the validation process is unsuitable for humans due to its safety profile and the lack of evidence-based studies regarding its potential harm. In fact, only a few formulations worldwide have incorporated n-propanol for hand antisepsis.

Given the fact that other properties of the formulations recommended by the WHO, such as their excellent tolerability, good acceptance among healthcare workers and low costs, are of great importance for a lasting clinical effect, the above results are considered acceptable and, according to the agreement of the WHO expert group, the two preparations can be used for surgical preparation. Institutions that choose to use WHO-recommended surgical hand preparation formulations should ensure that at least three, if not more, applications are used for a period of 3 to 5 minutes. For surgical procedures lasting more than 2 hours, surgeons should ideally practice a second-hand rub of approximately 1 minute, although further investigation is required on this aspect.

Cleaning and disinfection process for reusable hand rub bottles:

1. Move the empty bottle to the center point for reprocessing using standard operating protocols.

2. Wash the bottles thoroughly with detergent and tap water to remove any liquid residue.

3. If heat resistant, disinfect bottles thermally by boiling them in water. Whenever possible, thermal disinfection should be preferred to chemical disinfection. The latter increases costs and may introduce additional steps to wash away the remaining disinfectant. For chemical disinfection, soak the bottle in a 1000 ppm chlorine solution for at least 15 minutes, then rinse with sterile/chilled boiling water.

4. After thermal or chemical disinfection, let the bottles dry upside down in a bottle rack. Dry bottles should be closed with lids and protected from dust until use.

WHAT INGREDIENTS DO YOU REQUIRE TO MAKE HAND DISINFECTANTS?

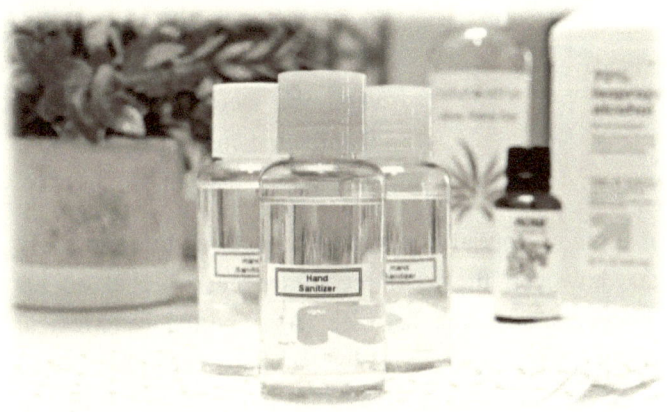

Hand disinfectants can be made at home using three main ingredients: isopropyl alcohol (91 percent or more), aloe vera gel, and a few drops of essential oil. Before you put all of these ingredients together, there are a few things you should know. Isopropyl alcohol is the main ingredient of disinfection in this DIY hand disinfection recipe. Use alcohol with an alcohol content of 91 percent or more to make your home disinfectant as effective as possible. Ideally, 99 percent is the best thing you can do, but anything over 91 still works efficiently to kill germs and bacteria.

Aloe vera gel is accessible in most stores and (now ...) online. Also, if you have aloe vera plants, you can cut leaves from the plants and use

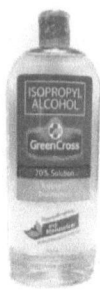

them for their healing (and disinfecting) properties. It is also vital for the recipe because of its moisturizing properties. It prevents your skin from drying out. With the absence of aloe vera, the alcohol in this hand disinfection recipe would cause your skin to dry out.

Some essential oils can be used as disinfectants. By far, however, the most recommended essential oil for disinfectants is the tea tree. As reported by Medical News Today, tea tree oil has antibacterial properties as well as anti-inflammatory, antifungal, and antiviral properties. While research is limited on which viruses can successfully fight the tea tree essential oil, it is believed to fight off the pathogens associated with acne, staphylococci, micrococci, Enterococcus faecalis, and

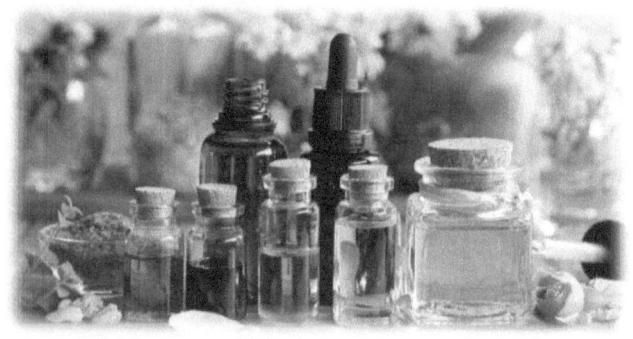

Pseudomonas aeruginosa. Cinnamon is another suggested essential oil for making hand sanitizers.

Cinnamon effectively "deactivated" the viral elements in some organisms. If you're just looking for a hand sanitizer that smells good, use lemon, orange, peppermint, or lavender. No matter which essential oil you choose, 8-15 drops should do the trick.

In addition to these three major ingredients, you will likely need a mixing bowl, spoon, measuring cup, and funnel. These things are not * necessary *, but they definitely make the measuring and cleaning process considerably easier!

HOW TO MAKE DIY HAND SANITIZER

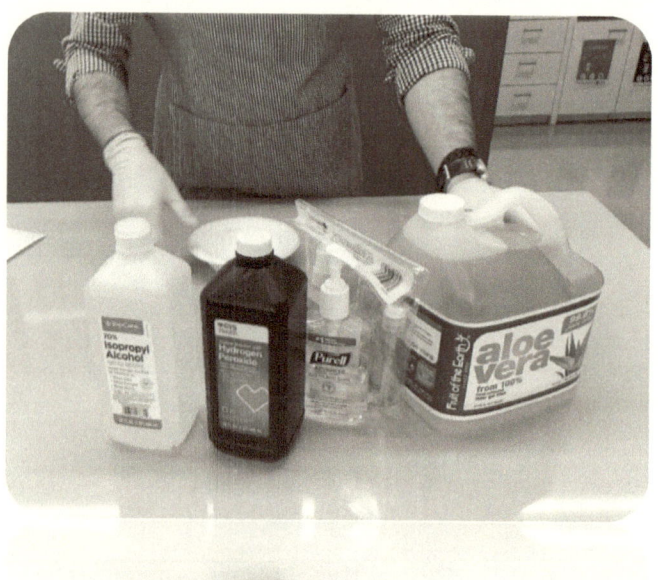

As the Flu continues to spread, the disease control centers have recommended "social distancing" and self-isolation whenever possible. And as you may have noticed, a side effect is that things are flying off the shelves at your local grocery store. One of these things? Hand disinfectant. Times are certainly desperate, but as you stock up on non-perishable goods, medication, and other important things that you may need in the next few weeks, consider what everyone will be consuming next - alcohol, aloe vera, and ethereal Oils - and be one step ahead of the game. While people are figuring out (namely googling) how to make their own disinfectant at home - remember, hand sanitizer was the first thing people were looking for during the initial Influenza threat! -Isopropyl alcohol, essential oils, and aloe vera gel are definitely the next goals of the people. If you've been looking for DIY hand sanitizers, here's what you need to know - from myths to facts to a professional's opinion of how to make it yourself. How to make your own disinfectant wipes at home during the flu virus crisis. How to make hand sanitizer.

It's all about the relationship, the ratio you need for the most effective hand sanitizer depends on the percentage of alcohol you use. For example, if you use isopropyl alcohol, which is 91 percent, you want a ratio of 3: 2, 3 tablespoons of alcohol to tablespoons of aloe. If you use 99 percent isopropyl alcohol, you want a 2: 1 ratio (3T alcohol, 1.5T aloe). Assuming you use 91 percent isopropyl alcohol, pour 1 cup into a mixing bowl. Next, add 2/3 cup of aloe vera gel. Add 8-15 drops of the essential oil of your choice. Mix everything with a spoon, then use a funnel to pump the mixture into a bottle. If you don't have a container with a pump, you can put your DIY hand sanitizer in a travel tube or one of those tiny salad dressing tubes that you put in the children's lunch! Alternatively, a spray bottle also works.

1 cup of Everclear

1/3 cup aloe vera

2 tablespoons of coconut oil

A few drops of essential oil

Hydrogen peroxide (quantity depends on supply)

Mix it in a bowl and portion it into a container.

What if you don't have aloe vera gel?

Don't worry; you can still make hand sanitizers without aloe vera gel. Just replace aloe vera with witch hazel. If you employ witch hazel as an alternative, the consistency of your disinfectant is more like a spray. For this reason, a spray bottle is probably best. If you are worried that your hands will dry out from alcohol, you can also add 1/4 teaspoon of vitamin E oil.

HOW TO DISINFECT AT HOME

Regular cleaning is one of the most active measures to combat Influenza and stop it from spreading. This includes washing hands, but also the regular disinfection of our houses. "According to the CDC guidelines, we should disinfect our house regularly," explains Gandhi. "In the first

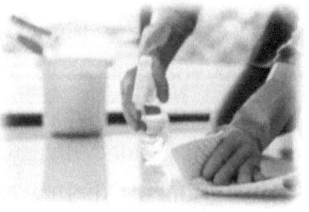

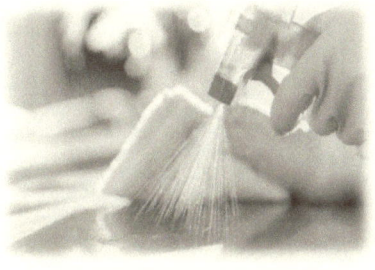

place, repeated hand washing for more than 20 seconds is the key. Use disposable gloves and wipe the surfaces with disinfectant or water and soap. You want to wipe tables, doorknobs, light switches, countertops, handles, desks, phones, keys, toilets, and sinks. "

What is the most effective way to wipe these surfaces? "You can also apply 70% alcohol to wipe surfaces," added Gandhi. "You can make a bleaching solution with 5T of bleach and 1 gallon of water. Honestly, if you don't have alcohol or bleach, I wouldn't

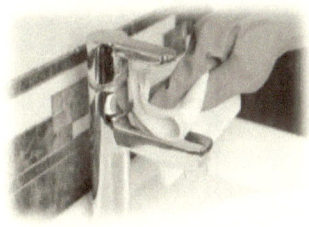

recommend making anything with vinegar or baking soda for disinfection. "However, the most important prevention tactic of all could only be social distancing." Social distancing is very important. Remember that our current health system does not have the effects of all people who are ill at the same time can endure. This is because we can stop the virus from spreading and relieve our current health system. "

HAND HYGIENE

Hand hygiene control is just the first step. Policies will now be in effect to render individuals accountable for the protection of paws.

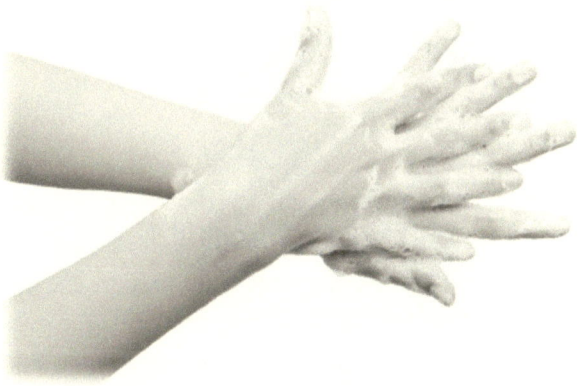

Hands play a significant role in infection transfer in healthcare settings, in manufacturing areas such as the food industry and even in the population and the home. No focus should be put on the significance of hand grooming in the prevention of infection. The value of hand hygiene for managing the transmission of infectious diseases is evident in the growing number of scientific literature publications in recent years, including significant hand hygienic papers in influential general medical journals. The goal of hand hygiene practices is to eliminate transient (contaminating) flora as rapidly as possible and to provide sustained antimicrobial activity on the resident flora. This means decontaminating the hands of temporary flora before the next touch in the sense of a healthcare setting. The sustained operation of the hand hygiene preparations during usage is particularly significant in health care environments where clean hands for longer periods of time are needed.

HAND CREAMS AND EMOLLIENTS

Sore, dry hands are a widely recorded issue among HCWs who sometimes have to wash their hands or decontaminate them. Lipids contribute to skin and skin cream barrier functions, lotions and emollients can boost skin hydration and thereby increase skin defense. A randomized, double-blind study of a barrier cream and an oil-based lotion found that the intended usage of both treatments significantly covered the hands of certain HCWs who had serious skin discomfort already. The same research found that skin development was correlated with increased washing of the hands. If barrier creams make a significant contribution to the overall avoidance of skin issues is not yet understood. Oil products can also impair the barrier role of latex gloves and the efficacy of antimicrobial agents used in hand hygiene.

RINGS

There are more micro-organisms beneath the skin than contact points. With the number of rings carried, the amount of micro-organisms decreases. Multivariate research in one report indicated that wearing rings is a significant risk factor for the transport of gram-negative bacilli, and S. Aureus on hands are also essential pathogens. There is also proof that animals trapped under the rings may be stored over many months. Handwashing was marginally less effective in an experimental model utilizing food handlers as participants in ring wearers, but it was in hands that were chemically polluted not under real-life circumstances. There is no evidence that hand washing is inefficient in-ring carriers, with most studies finding comparable bacterial numbers in-ring carriers and non-ring carriers. The possession of rings provides no justification for medical results, such as the prevalence of nosocomial illness.

WRISTWATCHES AND BRACELETS

It seems clear that hand hygiene procedures can not be sufficient in therapeutic areas where a wristwatch or bracelet is worn. Most recommendations on hospital infection control suggest the elimination of wristwatches and bracelets while exercising hand hygiene. A 'hygiene' and 'wristwatches' review on Medline only revealed two quotes concerning the hygiene of the hand and no quote using 'bracelet' and 'hygiene' as keywords. Research by 20 volunteers and 20 non-clinical volunteers showed that the skin under a wristwatch had become more colonized with micro-organisms than control sites with the skin beneath the band. Micro-organisms were unlikely to induce infection in a normal dental setting, but nosocomial pathogens were identified. However, the suggestion to not wear a wristwatch and enforcement is poorly backed by almost no other facts.

SLEEVES AND CUFFS

Arm hygiene legislation suggests rolling sleeves before personal hygiene procedures. Many uniform regulations often prescribe short sleeves, although, for HCWs who do not wear uniforms, short sleeves are not typically enforced. Wet sleeves, like any wet surface, may be assumed to function as a repository for micro-organisms that could be passed to hands through direct touch. The obvious macroscopic pollution of the mane during usual wear highlights their capacity for pathogen transmission. However, there is little proof in the scientific literature to endorse short sleeves.

FINGERNAILS, NAIL TECHNOLOGY, AND NAIL POLISH

The 0subungual area includes vast concentrations of bacteria that are relatively unavailable to the individual during hygiene procedures, rendering it impossible to cleanse relatively to the rest of the hands. This makes it easy to disinfect, though, it has also been found that longer nails have an improvement in the amount of the micro-organisms. More and more artificial nails are documented to be able to spread pathogens in the medical community. Artificial nails are more likely than human nails to be colonized with gram-negative bacilli and yeasts. In one analysis, the overall amount of species was not significant, whereas artificial nails were more likely to be colonized with Gram-negative bacteria and yeasts. The longer the nails were kept, the more often the pathogenes were extracted. There are proofs that washing artificial nails is not as successful as washing natural nails. Research comparing soap or alcohol gel in hand hygiene showed that HCWs with artificial nails have more bacteria than normal nails.

Works Cited

(n.d.). Retrieved from https://www.usp.org/sites/default/files/usp/document/about/public-policy/usp-co_vi_d19-handrub.pdf

e-liquid-recipes. (n.d.). Retrieved from DIY Hand Sanitizer / Disinfectant Recipes: https://e-liquid-recipes.com/handsanitizer

MCEVOY, S. D. (n.d.). *jakartapost*. Retrieved from https://www.thejakartapost.com/life/2020/03/24/homemade-hand-sanitizer-recipes-that-could-help-protect-against-flu virus.html

Rita Babeluk. Sabrina Jutz. Sarah Mertlitz, Johannes Matiase, and Christoph Klaus. (n.d.). *plosone*. Retrieved from https://journals.plos.org/plosone/article/file?type=printable&id=10.1371/journal.pone.0111969

Rogers, K. (2020, Feb 20). Retrieved from Encyclopaedia Britannica: https://www.britannica.com/science/science

USP-NF. (n.d.). *USP-NF*. Retrieved from https://www.usp.org/sites/default/files/usp/document/about/public-policy/usp-co_vi_d19-handrub.pdf

WHO. (n.d.). Retrieved from
https://www.who.int/gpsc/5may/Guide_to_Local_Prod
uction.pdf

Wilson, D. R. (n.d.). *How to Make Your Own Hand Sanitizer*. Retrieved from Healthline:
https://www.healthline.com/health/how-to-make-
hand-sanitizer